Thyroid Diet

How to Improve Thyroid Disorders, Manage Thyroid Symptoms, Lose Weight, and Improve Your Metabolism through Diet!

Table Of Contents

Introduction 1
Chapter 1: The Thyroid and its Common Disorders 2
Chapter 2: Importance of Iodine 7
Chapter 3: Foods to Avoid 12
Chapter 4: Other Nutrients for Thyroid Health 14
Chapter 5: Tips on Planning a Thyroid-Friendly Diet 21
Chapter 6: Natural Thyroid Solutions 25
Chapter 7: Recipes For Thyroid Health 28
Chapter 8: The Best Foods For Thyroid Health 34
Chapter 9: Vital Nutrients For Thyroid Health 37
Chapter 10: How Thyroid Disorders Are Diagnosed 40
Chapter 11: Medical Treatments For Thyroid Disorders 43
Chapter 12: How The Thyroid Works & Affects The Whole Body 46
Conclusion 51

Introduction

I want to thank you and congratulate you for picking up the book, "Thyroid Diet: How to Improve Thyroid Disorders, Manage Thyroid Symptoms, Lose Weight, and Improve Your Metabolism through Diet!".

This is the recently updated 2nd edition. This new edition has been updated with a range of new information, making this a complete guide to thyroid disorders and improving them with diet!

This book contains helpful information about thyroid disorders, and how they can be improved through dietary changes, medicines, and other methods.

You will soon learn about the different thyroid disorders that people suffer from, their causes, and also how to improve and prevent them.

Thyroid disorders are primarily the result of dietary insufficiencies, and as such this book will be focusing on diet. You will soon discover the different foods that cause thyroid disorders, along with those that help to prevent and cure them.

This book will explain to you tips and techniques that will allow you to begin successfully managing and recovering from your thyroid disorder with the help of food! By making the simple dietary changes suggested within this guide, you'll be able to improve your thyroid disorder, or potentially prevent yourself from developing one in the first place!

Thanks again for taking the time to read this book, I hope you enjoy it!

Chapter 1:
The Thyroid and its Common Disorders

The thyroid is one of the body's endocrine glands. It is found in the neck area, below the Adam's apple and just in front of the trachea. It has a butterfly-like shape with the left and right lobes linked together by a narrow gland tissue in the middle called an isthmus.

The thyroid produces a number of thyroid hormones that influence the body's metabolism, protein generation, internal temperature, and holistic development. The two main thyroid hormones produced are triiodothyronine (T_3) and thyroxine (T_4), which is also sometimes called tetraiodothyronine. Sufficient thyroid hormone generation is vital for brain development, especially of infants and children. It is also essential for prenatal development as adequate maternal thyroid hormones (hormones coming from the mother) are needed to protect the fetus from any neurodevelopmental disorders.

With all of these important functions, it is clear that the thyroid is one of the most essential organs of the human body. And like all the other organs, the thyroid is not immune from illnesses and disorders that specifically affect it.

The most common types of thyroid disorders are the following:

1. Goiter – is the conventional term used for the enlargement of the thyroid gland. There are many causes of thyroid swelling, but statistics show that more than 90 percent of goiters around the world are caused by iodine deficiency. Other possible causes of goiter are congenital hypothyroidism, repeated intake of goitrogens (foods that suppress the absorption of iodine by the body), Basedow syndrome (more popularly known as Graves' disease), Hashimoto's thyroiditis, pituitary gland disease, and adverse reactions to drugs or other medications.

Not all cases of goiter may show any symptoms, although the typical ones are a noticeable bulging of the neck, having a hard time breathing or swallowing, a firm feeling around the throat, coughing, and sometimes huskiness of voice.

Treatment for goiters varies depending on the root cause. Some benign goiters that have only mild swelling are usually not treated at all and are allowed to heal on their own. With the addition of more iodine in the standard, everyday diet, particularly with the increased availability of iodized salt, the incidence of goiter worldwide has significantly gone down over the years.

2. Hyperthyroidism – is a disorder in which the thyroid gland excessively produces thyroid hormones that are no longer needed by the body. This overproduction is a problem, because when there is an abundance of T_3 and T_4 hormones in the body, its metabolism is drastically stimulated. This makes a person lose weight rapidly, sometimes dangerously, and causes them to experience abnormal sweating, irregular heartbeat, and anxiety attacks.

The common causes of hyperthyroidism are iodine oversufficiency, swelling of the thyroid gland that leaks out excess thyroid hormones, tumors in the testes (for men) or ovary (for women), and the over consumption of tetraiodothyronine (T_4 hormones) found in dietary supplements or medicines that are prescribed to treat hypothyroidism.

This condition is somewhat difficult to diagnose as most of its major symptoms are also common to other diseases, such as abrupt weight loss, rapid heartbeat (typically over a hundred beats per minute), heart palpitations, frequent mood swings, anxiousness, shaking of the hands and fingers, increased sweating, insomnia, tiredness and weariness, and thinning of the hair and skin. Most of the time, though, there are no symptoms at all, which is another reason why it is hard to detect this kind of thyroid disorder.

Fortunately, there are dietary treatments to improve the symptoms of hyperthyroidism. Consuming the right amounts of calories, sodium, vitamins, minerals, and other nutrients could help prevent the production of too much thyroid hormones in the body.

3. Hypothyroidism – is the exact opposite of hyperthyroidism as it is the condition when the thyroid gland does not produce enough thyroid hormones for the body to utilize. Again, this other extreme is a problem because without enough T_3 and T_4 hormones in the system, the body's metabolism becomes too slow. It results in weight gain, fatigue, physical and mental weaknesses, and sometimes depression.

For little children, insufficient thyroid hormones critically affect physical growth and intellectual development, which could sometimes lead to cretinism. Prolonged and untreated hypothyroidism could also cause other kinds of conditions and illnesses such as peripheral neuropathy, heart disease, myxedema, infertility, and some mental disorders.

This inadequate production of thyroid hormones is typically caused by treatments and medications for hyperthyroidism, treatments and medications for heart diseases and mental disorders, the complete or partial removal of the thyroid gland via surgery to remove cancer, and having insufficient iodine in the diet.

Similar to other thyroid disorders, one of the most effective ways of alleviating the symptoms of hypothyroidism is by having proper food and nutritional intake as well.

4. Thyroid Cancer – This is one of the rarest forms of cancers and is normally treatable. It is easily curable because its onset is easy to detect. There are also many effective remedies available today. However, it can still recur even after a lot of years of successful treatment.

Medical experts and practitioners still cannot pinpoint the exact causes of thyroid cancer. However, it is widely speculated to be the result of DNA changes brought about by old age. It could also be genetic or hereditary in nature. It is also observed that people who have been subjected to a lot of past radiation therapies in the chest, neck, and head, have a higher risk of obtaining thyroid cancer later on in their lives.

The common symptoms are a noticeable bump in the neck, soreness of the neck and the inner ears, difficulty in breathing and swallowing, huskiness of voice, and recurrent coughing that is unrelated to ordinary flu, cold, or any lung disease.

The conventional treatments for thyroid cancer are surgery and radiation therapy, although having the right diet could also help in relieving its symptoms.

5. Thyroiditis – is a term used to refer to a wide array of conditions that cause the inflammation of the thyroid gland. The common causes of inflammation are either an autoimmune disorder or a viral disease that specifically attacks the thyroid.

Similar to hyperthyroidism, thyroiditis' symptoms are also the signs and symptoms of other common diseases. This is why it takes a few more tests before it can be diagnosed correctly. Some of these indications are tiredness, weight gain, nausea, depression, drying of the skin, and infrequent bowel movement. In extreme cases, the inflammation of the thyroid causes the body temperature to drop, the areas around the eyes to become puffy, and the heart rate to become very slow which may continue to the point of failing.

Treatments are given to a patient according to what kind of thyroiditis they're suffering from. Among the treatment options are surgery, and the taking of antibiotics or other medications. Consuming the right amounts of the recommended foods could also help a lot in preventing the acquisition of this disease.

Managing Thyroid Disorders using Proper Diet

Your food intake can affect the health and function of your thyroid more than you may know. That is why it is necessary to watch what you eat in order to keep your thyroid gland in peak condition.

The next chapters will talk more about the foods to eat, foods to avoid, and how to plan the right diet to help treat and prevent each of the common thyroid disorders mentioned above.

Chapter 2:
Importance of Iodine

An insufficiency of iodine in the diet is the number one cause of basically all types of thyroid disorders. This is especially true in poor nations where a significant shortage in food supply is always experienced. Thus, its citizens are not conscious of, or are not interested in, consuming a proper diet. However, in countries where there is more awareness, and iodized salt is cheap and readily available in the market, cases of thyroid disorders are actually very low.

Importance of Iodine

Iodine in the blood is taken by the thyroid gland in order to activate the process of producing thyroid hormones. When there is not enough iodine in the bloodstream, another endocrine gland called the pituitary gland (found in the brain) communicates to the rest of the body that there is a said insufficiency. When this happens, the pituitary gland releases a hormone called Thyroid-Stimulating Hormone, or TSH, which forces the thyroid gland to produce more T_3 and T_4 hormones. This is harmful because it causes the thyroid gland to become enlarged or swollen, which then causes different kinds of thyroid problems.

Therefore, it is highly important to have sufficient iodine in the body for the general health and strength of the thyroid gland. The recommended daily intake of iodine is 150 micrograms.

To give you an idea of the proper amount and the right kinds of food to eat to prevent iodine deficiency, below is a list of iodine-rich foods.

List of Iodine-rich Foods

Aside from regularly using iodized salt in preparing your meals, here are some foods that you may incorporate in your daily diet in order for you to increase your iodine intake:

1. Milk – although this beverage is more popular for providing your body with the essential nutrients of vitamin D and calcium, it is actually a significant source of iodine as well. A glass of milk includes 56 micrograms of iodine, which is around 37 percent of the total recommended daily intake. Other dairy products such as organic cheese and yogurt are also high in iodine.

2. Yogurt – a cup of plain yogurt has about 150 micrograms of iodine, which is 100 percent of the recommended daily consumption. Having yogurt every morning for breakfast is a good idea as it also provides a healthy dose of protein and calcium.

3. Cheddar cheese – an ounce of this type of cheese provides approximately 12 micrograms of iodine. The portion should be quite small, as the ounce serving contains 452 calories. Still, it is still a nice option to consider for cheese lovers.

4. Potatoes – this root crop is another abundant source of iodine. A regular medium-sized potato contains a whopping 60 micrograms of iodine. Preparing it baked or boiled is better than mashing it, as most of the dietary benefits of potatoes, such as potassium, vitamins, and fiber, are held in their skin. It is also better to only consume the organic kind, since the skin

of potatoes keep much of the pesticides used during its farming.

5. Hard-boiled egg – a large-sized hard-boiled egg can provide around 12 micrograms of iodine, or a little less than 10 percent of the recommended daily intake. Aside from that, eggs are also good antioxidants. They provide fair amounts of calcium, zinc, and vitamins D and A.

6. White pea bean – beans are generally good sources of iodine, but white pea beans have been found to be the most iodine-rich. A half cup of these beans will give you around 32 micrograms of iodine. Apart from that, they also contains high amounts of fiber that aids proper digestion. Also, unlike other canned products that normally lose their dietary values because of processing, canned white pea beans retain most of their nutrients even when processed or canned.

7. Cranberries – aside from being an effective antioxidant, cranberries are also a rich source of iodine. A single ounce of fresh cranberries has about 100 micrograms of iodine, which is almost the amount required for the recommended daily consumption. Cranberries provide moderate amounts of fiber, vitamin C, and manganese, and are also a rich source of phytochemicals that boost the cardiovascular and immune systems. Cranberry juice is also famous for being effective in preventing urinary tract infections. They are actually considered by most dieticians as one of the world's healthiest foods.

8. Strawberries – another fruit that contains a fairly good amount of iodine is the strawberry. One cup of fresh strawberries can give you about 15 micrograms of

iodine, exactly 10 percent of the recommended daily intake. Like cranberries, they are also a rich source of vitamin C, manganese, and phytochemicals.

9. Shrimp – as with all the other seafood, shrimps are a good source of iodine as well. A three-ounce portion contains 35 micrograms of iodine, or 23 percent of the recommended daily consumption. It can also provide sufficient amounts of calcium, protein, and omega 3 fatty acids. Shrimps are also deemed beneficial to the circulatory system as they enhance the proportion of LDL and HDL cholesterol levels and significantly reduce triglycerides.

10. Lobster – lobsters are also great sources of iodine as a 100-gram portion of it has 100 micrograms of iodine, or 67 percent of the recommended daily intake. They are also rich in iron, zinc, phosphorus, potassium, magnesium, calcium, and vitamins A, B2, B3, B6, and B12.

11. Tuna – this saltwater fish is rich in iodine and is an important source of omega 3 fatty acids as well. It contains 34 micrograms of iodine for every six ounce serving. When it comes to canned tuna, those that are prepared in oil have more iodine than those prepared in water. The other nutrients sufficiently provided by tuna are iron, protein, and vitamin D.

12. Cod – another saltwater fish that contains huge amounts of iodine is cod. Just a three-ounce portion has an incredible 99 micrograms of iodine, or about 66 percent of the recommended daily intake. Aside from that, cod liver oil also provides sufficient amounts of omega 3 fatty acids and vitamins A, D, and E.

13. Kelp – is a large seaweed found in the shallow parts of the ocean. Its iodine content is enormous. Just a mere quarter of an ounce contains 4,500 micrograms of iodine, which is 3,000 percent of the recommended daily intake. It is advised to eat only small servings at a time as it may result in an oversufficiency of iodine. Other species of kelp that have high concentrations of iodine are wakame (80 micrograms per tablespoon), arame (730 micrograms per tablespoon), hiziki (780 micrograms per tablespoon), and kombu (1,450 micrograms in every 1-inch portion).

14. Turkey meat – apart from having the most protein content for every ounce among all meats, it is also a good source of iodine. Three ounces contains 34 micrograms of iodine. It also gives a healthy dose of potassium, phosphorus, and B vitamins.

These are only some of the foods that are rich in iodine, and there are many more. It is also important to keep in mind, however, that the overconsumption of iodine is also not good for your thyroid health, which is why a balanced diet is needed.

Chapter 3:
Foods to Avoid

If there are food items that can improve the function of the thyroid gland, there are also certain food types that specifically contribute to its dysfunction. These food types should thus be avoided as much as possible. Some of these foods impede the thyroid's ability to get iodine from the blood, while others prevent the production of thyroid hormones itself. Either way, both are not useful to help keep the thyroid healthy and functioning properly. Below are some of the food products to avoid if you have a thyroid disorder.

1. Cruciferous vegetables such as cauliflower, broccoli, kale, Brussel sprouts, turnip, and cabbage. It is said that these veggies inhibit the absorption of iodine by the thyroid gland. It is not advised, however, to totally eliminate them from your diet as they do provide a lot of health benefits as well. To remove their anti-iodine effect on the body, simply shred or boil them before eating.

2. Any soy products such as soy beans, soy sauce, soy milk, and tofu. A study issued by the National Institutes of Health said that soy products have anti-thyroid characteristics that are intensified when a person is already suffering from an iodine deficiency. However, as long as you are eating enough iodine-rich foods, you can still consume these products for their specific dietary benefits, but in small amounts only.

3. Processed foods such as white sugar, white flour, and white bread.

4. Artificial sweeteners such as aspartame. Medical experts say that the regular consumption of aspartame leads to autoimmune diseases that affect the thyroid.

5. Gluten contained in wheat, barley, and rye, as well as in all processed foods. It is reported that it also causes autoimmune conditions that induce thyroid swelling.

6. Any fried or greasy food. Meats that are fatty, such as pork and beef, should also be avoided. Opt for friendlier sources of protein instead, like lentils, beans, milk, eggs, fish and other seafood.

7. Coffee, tea, soda, and other caffeinated products. You can consume them daily but only in small amounts.

8. Alcoholic drinks of any kind.

Since thyroid problems are most often caused by iodine deficiency, its prevention (as well as treatment if you already have it) begins by making sure that you have enough iodine in your daily food intake. This should be done in tandem with staying away from foods that lower its effectiveness.

Chapter 4:
Other Nutrients for Thyroid Health

As you may have already presumed, iodine is definitely not the only nutrient that can help to improve thyroid disorders. Although it is the main nutrient that the body needs to maintain good thyroid health, there are also other nutrients that support the thyroid gland and allow it to function well. Below are some of these nutrients and the most common food products that contain them.

1. **Selenium** – apart from iodine, selenium is considered as the most essential element for thyroid health. It helps the thyroid gland by regulating the production of thyroid hormones and the reusing of the body's excess iodine. It also benefits all of the body cells that specifically utilize thyroid hormones by converting thyroxine (T4) into the more active triiodothyronine (T3) for better metabolism function. Selenium also relieves social, chemical, and oxidative stress experienced by the thyroid.

   Without enough selenium in the body, the thyroid works in a constant state of stress, which could eventually break it down, making it detrimental to a person's overall wellbeing. Hypothyroidism is one of the major effects of insufficient selenium. Other effects include tiredness, depression, intellectual disability, cretinism for infants, and frequent miscarriages for women. Other diseases that come from selenium deficiency are Kashin-Beck disease and Keshan disease.

   Common selenium-rich foods are Brazil nuts, tuna, halibut, snapper, cod, shrimp, clams, oysters, sunflower seeds, whole grains, whole-wheat bread, and shitake and button mushrooms.

According to the World Health Organization (WHO), the recommended daily intake of selenium is 70 to 350 micrograms per day. Consuming too much of it (around 40 times of the recommended) is considered toxic.

2. **Iron** – This is the first of three trace metals that are considered as essential nutrients for thyroid health. All of the body's cells need iron to carry oxygen to its different parts, and also to store oxygen in the muscles. When it comes to the thyroid gland, iron helps in the production of thyroid hormones as well.

Iron-deficiency anemia, or not having enough iron in the blood, affects the efficacy of iodine in the body's systems. This reduces the performance of the thyroid. Iodine and iron work together to provide a steady balance in synthesizing thyroid hormones. Other effects of a lack of iron in the body are dizziness, fatigue, heart palpitations, irritability, cramping, hand numbness, diarrhea, loss of sex drive, and loss of appetite.

Foods that have high amounts of iron are seafood, poultry, red meat, dried fruit, peanuts, cashew nuts, almonds, lentils, white beans, and dark green leafy vegetables such as spinach, lettuce, cabbage, collard greens, mustard greens, and turnip greens.

The recommended daily allowance for iron varies from 7 to 27 milligrams a day, depending on age. Pregnant or breastfeeding mothers will also have a different requirement for iron intake.

3. **Zinc** – your thyroid also needs this trace metal to function properly. Zinc helps the hypothalamus, which is the part of the brain that connects the nervous system to the endocrine system, to produce Thyrotropin-Releasing Hormone or TRH. TRH triggers the pituitary gland's production of TSH (Thyroid-Stimulating Hormone). This in turn helps the thyroid to release its T_3 and T_4 hormones.

   When there is insufficient zinc in the body, there is also not enough TRH. The thyroid becomes slow and is put under stress, which causes hypothyroidism. However, when there is too much zinc in the body, the thyroid becomes too active, causing hyperthyroidism. The key is to only consume the right amount of zinc in your diet.

   Zinc is commonly found in oysters, portabella and shitake mushrooms, lean pork, lean poultry, beef, lamb, spinach, beans, pumpkin seeds, squash seeds, cashew nuts, and dark chocolate and cocoa.

   The recommended daily consumption is 3 to 40 milligrams per day. This recommended value could vary depending on age and whether a woman is pregnant or breastfeeding.

4. **Copper** – lastly, the third trace metal that the thyroid needs besides iron and zinc is copper. The relationship of copper with the thyroid gland is associated with zinc. This is because as an individual consumes more zinc in their diet, the copper levels in the body are reduced. This, of course, is not good. Copper provides many health benefits such as balancing the body's estrogen and progesterone levels, and regulating calcium in the vascular system to promote nutrient absorption.

On its own, copper is also good for the thyroid as it keeps the body from accumulating excess T_4 hormones in the bloodstream. It also keeps the thyroid healthy by controlling the release of thyroid hormones.

Common sources of copper are squid, octopus, crabs, lobsters, shrimps, oysters, shitake mushroom, chickpeas, kidney beans, sesame seeds, kale, avocadoes, and prunes and other dried fruits such as figs, apricots, and peaches.

It is recommended that about 340 to 1,000 micrograms of copper be consumed by the average individual per day. More than that is considered toxic.

5. **Vitamins A, C, and E** – these are antioxidant vitamins that help alleviate oxidative stress which can fatally affect the thyroid. Oxidative stress is perhaps the main reason for the development of many types of cancers, including thyroid cancer, and is also the main cause of Graves' disease, which is the most common type of hyperthyroidism. Antioxidants fight oxidation and the release of free radicals in the body.

Foods that contain vitamin A are spinach, kale, asparagus, lettuce, carrots, winter squash, sweet potatoes, and animal liver. Some vitamin C-rich foods are citrus fruits, tomatoes, papaya, strawberries, kiwi, guava, chili peppers, red bell peppers, green bell peppers, and kale. For vitamin E, the foods recommended are dark leafy vegetables, asparagus, beans, animal liver, almonds, peanuts, and sunflower seeds.

Recommended daily allowances for each are: vitamin A – 600 micrograms per day; vitamin C – 75 milligrams per day; and vitamin E – 10 milligrams per day.

6. **B vitamins** – the eight B vitamins are thiamin, riboflavin, niacin, pantothenic acid, pyridoxine, biotin, folate, and cobalamin. They are marked by the symbols B_1, B_2, B_3, B_5, B_6, B_7, B_9, and B_{12} respectively. They play a great role when it comes to proper cell metabolism. For the thyroid, B vitamins assist in the production of healthy and sufficient thyroid hormones, particularly T_4.

   Foods that are high in B vitamins are:

   - thiamin – dark green leafy vegetables, whole grain cereals

   - riboflavin – milk, yogurt, cheese

   - niacin – eggs, chicken, turkey, salmon, tuna, legumes, peanuts

   - pantothenic acid and biotin – animal liver, egg yolks, salmon, avocado

   - pyridoxine – seafood, poultry, dark green leafy vegetables, bananas, potatoes

   - folate – grains, rice, spinach, turnip greens, fresh fruits and vegetables

   - cobalamin – soy products, clams, mussels, crabs, beef

The recommended daily values for each B vitamin are:

- thiamin – 1.4 milligrams per day
- riboflavin – 1.2 milligrams per day
- niacin – 18 milligrams per day
- pantothenic acid – 6 milligrams per day
- pyridoxine – 2 milligrams per day
- biotin – 30 micrograms per day
- folate – 400 micrograms per day
- cobalamin – 6 micrograms per day

7. **Omega 3 fatty acids** – although there are still no official reports, medical experts are currently looking closely at the possible ways in which this polyunsaturated fatty acid improves thyroid conditions.

Fatty acids are essential to health as they are the main part of cell membranes. They also help in promoting proper cell growth, controlling inflammation, and relieving autoimmune diseases, such as many types of thyroiditis. This means that if a person has a thyroid condition that is autoimmune in nature, and they don't consume enough omega 3 in their diet, then the thyroid may go haywire.

Since the body cannot create omega 3 fatty acids on its own, it has to be taken through the person's diet. The major source of this nutrient is fish oil and seafood.

There is no recommended daily dosage for omega 3 fatty acid, although supplements are advised by most doctors.

Chapter 5:
Tips on Planning a Thyroid-Friendly Diet

A thyroid-friendly diet is so much more important than a weight loss diet. It is something that is needed to improve thyroid disorders, manage their symptoms, and improve proper metabolism. Moreover, it is not just about knowing what and what not to eat, but also knowing *how* and *how much* to eat.

Weight Loss and Gain

It is important to note that weight loss and weight gain are the common symptoms of hyperthyroidism and hypothyroidism, and not their causes. You don't get thyroid disorders from losing or gaining weight. When you have fewer thyroid hormones, your body burns lesser calories, which promotes weight gain. In contrast, excessive thyroid hormones tend to accelerate the metabolism, which makes you lose weight. It is important to consider these factors when planning your own diet.

The right diet for people with different thyroid disorders consists mostly of the same types of foods, only with different amounts or servings depending if one has excessive thyroid hormones (hyperthyroidism) or insufficient thyroid hormones (hypothyroidism).

In any case, however, a thyroid-friendly diet is really quite the same as that of what a normal person should be eating to stay healthy. It is always necessary to incorporate more fruits and vegetables in the diet, and have less sugar, caffeine, fatty foods, and processed foods.

Below are some tips on how to plan a thyroid-friendly diet:

1. Find the Right Substitutes

All types of diets basically want to cut down on sugar, caffeine, harmful fat, and processed foods. These same elements are especially detrimental for someone with a thyroid disorder. There are many ways to cut down on these damaging foods without torturing yourself. For example, if you have a really sweet tooth, then you can try a piece of fresh fruit or berries with whipped cream as a substitute for cake or other pastries. You can still have the same sweet flavor, but with more fresh food included in the serving.

2. Have as much Antioxidants as possible

If you are managing an autoimmune form of thyroid disorder, like Hashimoto's disease, you will need more antioxidants in your diet. Choose foods that are rich in vitamins A, C, and E, as these are great antioxidant vitamins, as mentioned in the previous chapter.

Dark green leafy vegetables (spinach, kale, arugula, lettuce, collards, and other greens), citrus fruits (oranges, grapefruit, lemon, lime, tangerine, and pomelo), and nuts and beans, should be the major components of your food intake. As mentioned in the previous chapter, antioxidants relieve oxidative stress that causes autoimmune thyroid conditions.

3. Organic is Better

As much as possible, it is better to eat organic food. For one, it contains lower amounts of chemicals, like insecticides, herbicides, and other forms of pesticides, that can further damage the thyroid. One of the major goals of a thyroid-friendly diet is to eliminate as much stress as possible from the thyroid gland, and organic foods are the best way to do this!

4. Keep Blood Sugar in Check

Erratic blood sugar fluctuations have a negative effect on the thyroid's physical properties. High blood sugar causes inflammation and swelling to the thyroid gland if not properly regulated. It is better to have six small meals of 300 calories in a day than have 3 large portions of 600 calories, for example. This is ideal, except for meals after strenuous workouts or activities, in which you need more carbohydrates to recover and compensate for the energy you have just burned.

5. Make Your Body More Alkaline

Cells function better in an alkaline environment rather than in an acidic one. On the other hand, an acidic system puts a lot of unnecessary stress on the body, leading to a slower metabolism and many deficiencies, including that of thyroid hormones. Too much alkalinity, however, is also not advised as the body may experience catabolism, where tissues and cells break down rapidly because of chemical stress. The ideal pH level of the body should be in between 6.5 to 7.5.

To have a more alkaline system, you simply have to include more fresh fruits and vegetables in your meals. Alkaline-inducing foods are those rich in calcium, zinc, potassium, and magnesium, such as carrots, eggplants, celery, cucumber, tomatoes, watercress, wheat grass, radishes, onions, kale, spinach, dandelions, rutabaga, sweet potatoes, and seaweeds.

Have smaller amounts of meat and dairy products because these protein-rich foods typically promote an acidic environment. However, eliminating protein completely from your diet will also have adverse effects on the thyroid, so it is important to find the right balance.

6. Consume Enough Protein

Speaking of protein, according to medical research, for each kilogram of body weight, an average person has to consume at least 800 milligrams of protein per day. However, this figure is not applicable for people who experience high stress levels. That is why 1.2 grams of protein per day is the most ideal for those who have thyroid conditions.

For best results, try to consume protein only from healthy sources such as fish, poultry, eggs, legumes, nuts, and organic dairy products.

7. Keep Yourself Hydrated

Water is the best friend of someone with a thyroid disorder. Not only does plain water support the optimal health of the thyroid gland, but it is also a great way to feel fuller whenever you get unhealthy food cravings. Water is also very good for preventing constipation, which is a common symptom of thyroid disorders. If you have to consume a beverage, your first choice should always be water.

8. Find the Right Balance

While there are foods that inhibit thyroid performance, such as cruciferous vegetables and soy products, it is important to keep in mind that they should not be completely taken away from a balanced diet. Consume them in moderation, and be sure to have enough thyroid-friendly foods in your diet to counter the negative effects.

Chapter 6:
Natural Thyroid Solutions

There are a number of natural thyroid solutions that you can rely on in order to improve your thyroid health. These include good nutrition, adequate exercise, and proper rest.

Your thyroid needs certain nutrients to let it carry out its functions properly. You should also make time for exercise to improve your blood flow and allow your thyroid hormones to work on all your cells, as well as rest. Getting proper rest is the best way for your body to recover after carrying out its various functions, including that of your thyroid.

The following are a few strategies for naturally improving your thyroid health:

1. Fruit up.

Incorporate more fruits as well as vegetables into your diet. It is best to eat the freshest local produce you can get your hands on, and make sure to choose organic vegetables and fruits that are in season. But know that even frozen vegetables and fruits are beneficial to your thyroid's health.

2. Spill the beans.

Your diet could benefit greatly from legumes and beans. These food items are rich sources of a number of minerals and vitamins that your thyroid gland needs to produce the thyroid hormones that your cells need to properly function. Moreover, legumes and beans provide you the protein your body needs, especially if you limit your intake of meat.

3. Try something fishy.

Increase your intake of fish for the sake of your thyroid's health. Besides being a lean source of protein and omega-3 fatty acids, fish is not difficult to incorporate in your dishes. Just make sure that you do not choose fish with a high mercury content, as it may worsen your thyroid problem.

4. Water it down.

Drinking lots of water is another way of improving the health of your thyroid. Staying hydrated is also an effective method of giving your general health a boost.

5. Keep it whole.

You will do your thyroid a great service by reducing your consumption of processed foods, particularly those which contain added sugar. As much as possible, eat only whole foods – unprocessed foods that have most of their nutrients intact. To simplify things, avoid any white food item: white pasta, white rice, and white bread. Choose whole grain pasta, brown rice, and whole grain bread to keep your thyroid in tip-top shape.

6. Choose lean and organic.

Reduce your intake of meat, especially red meats. If doing so is not possible, you just have to make sure that you are eating lean meats, grass-fed beef, and skinless poultry. You also have to ensure that you are consuming hormone-free and antibiotic-free meats, which you can get in the organic section at the supermarket.

7. Go sugar-free.

Limit your intake of sugar to ensure that your thyroid problem does not worsen. Keep your blood sugar levels down by consuming whole grains and other complex carbohydrates, and doing away with sugar (table sugar, corn syrup, and other form of simple sugar) as well as sugar substitutes. You may use stevia instead as a form of natural sweetener.

8. Work out.

Exercise plays an important role in improving the health of your thyroid. Make sure that you exercise for half an hour on a daily basis. You can take up something as simple as brisk walking. Simply speed things up or walk a bit longer if you want to take your exercise routine to the next level.

9. Say no to stress.

It helps your thyroid function properly if you take steps to decrease your stress levels. Determine what factors trigger your feelings of stress and then find ways to tone down their effects on your health. One way is to go easy on yourself is by learning how to relax through different meditation techniques (visualization and deep breathing).

10. Give it a rest.

It is important that you take the time to have proper rest. Treat your body to adequate sleep during nighttime, and make sure you get adequate rest in the daytime. Doing so will help your thyroid, which is highly sensitive and responsive to stress, avoid getting all worked up. Make sure you get all the rest and relaxation you can possibly get if your thyroid is in bad health.

Chapter 7:
Recipes For Thyroid Health

You can give your thyroid a hand by making sure that you eat meals that improve its health. The trick is to keep your meal choices varied enough that your palate will not feel limited or deprived. Consider following these recipes to get you started on having an improved thyroid function as well as a better state of health in general.

BREAKFAST: **Savory Green Plantain Pancakes**

Ingredients:

Coconut oil (1/4 cup)

Butter, divided (2 teaspoons)

Lime juice (1 tablespoon)

Green plantains (1 ½ pounds)

Sea salt (a few pinches)

For filling:

Coconut butter (2 tablespoons)

Vanilla essence (1 teaspoon)

Lime juice (1 teaspoon)

Berries, mixed (1 cup)

Sea salt (a pinch)

Directions:

1. Cut up the plantains into thick slices.

2. Place the sliced plantains in a food processor. Add the salt, coconut oil, and lime juice before blending until the mixture is smooth. Pour some water (about 1/8 cup) into the mixture to improve its consistency.

3. Heat a skillet over low-medium heat. Place one portion of the butter (1 teaspoon) on the skillet.

4. Once the butter is melted, add ½ of the plantain mixture. Allow the mixture to spread on the skillet.

5. Cover slightly to cook while letting the water evaporate. Cook for about ten minutes or until the pancake surface turns dry. Cook on the other side for two to three minutes or until golden-brown. Repeat the procedure with the remaining mixture.

6. Transfer the pancakes onto a serving dish. Meanwhile, place the ingredients for the filling in the food processor. Process until the filling mixture is well blended, and then pour on the pancakes.

7. Serve immediately.

LUNCH: **Pan-seared Chicken and Sautéed Vegetables**

Ingredients:

Coconut oil, for frying

Sea salt, cayenne, black pepper, paprika, and cumin

Chicken breasts, pastured (2 pieces)

<u>*For sautéed vegetables:*</u>

Cabbage, thinly sliced (1/4 head)

Olive oil, organic (2 teaspoons)

Leek, green, washed, chopped (1 piece)

Kale, thinly sliced (2 to 3 leaves)

Carrots, thinly sliced (2 pieces)

Water (1/3 cup)

Sea salt (a few pinches)

Directions:

1. To make the sautéed vegetables: Heat a sauté pan over medium-high heat. Pour the water into the pan. Add the cabbage, leeks, kale, and carrots. Cover the pan and steam for about two to three minutes. Remove the cover to allow the water to evaporate before drizzling with the olive oil. Season with the sea salt and toss well. Remove the pan from the heat and set aside.

2. Place the chicken breasts in a small bowl. Add the cayenne, sea salt, paprika, black pepper, and cumin and rub onto the meat.

3. Place a skillet over medium-high heat. Add the coconut oil. Once the oil is heated, add the chicken breasts. Cover and cook on every side for about three to four minutes. Remove from the pan and place on a platter.

4. Serve the chicken with the sautéed vegetables.

DINNER: **Baked Fish with Lemon and Herbs**

Ingredients:

Butter, thinly sliced (2 tablespoons)

Lemons, large, thinly sliced into rounds (2 pieces)

Dill (1 tablespoon)

Parsley (1 tablespoon)

Oregano (1 tablespoon)

Dover sole, filleted (1 pound)

Black pepper, freshly round (a dash)

Sea salt (a pinch)

Directions:

1. Set the oven at 375 degrees to preheat.
2. Line a baking pan (9x12") with parchment paper. Lay the fish fillets on the pan and sprinkle with black pepper and sea salt.
3. Top each of the fillets with dill, parsley, oregano, butter slices, and lemon slices.
4. Place in the oven to bake for about ten to twelve minutes or until the fillets are flaky and light.

SALAD: **Red Potato Salad**

Ingredients:

Sauerkraut, lacto-fermented, chopped (3/4 cup)

Vinegar, apple cider (2 tablespoons)

Bacon (4 strips)

Mayonnaise (3/4 cup)

Dijon mustard (2 tablespoons)

Red potatoes, unpeeled (2 pounds)

Spring onions, chopped (1/4 cup)

Sea salt (1 tablespoon)

Directions:

1. Set the oven at 350 degrees to preheat.
2. Fill a pot with water and mix in some salt. Add the potatoes and boil for forty-five minutes to let the potatoes soften.
3. Place the bacon in the oven and bake for 45 minutes or until golden-brown.
4. Remove the boiled potatoes from the pot. Let stand to cool before cutting into half-inch cubes.
5. Place the cubed potatoes in a large bowl. Gently fold in the chopped sauerkraut, apple cider vinegar, mayonnaise, mustard, sea salt, and spring onions.
6. Serve and enjoy.

SNACK: **Raisin Cinnamon Cookies**

Ingredients:

Raisins, yellow (1/4 cup)

Rice flour, white (1 ½ cups)

Baking powder (1 teaspoon)

Egg, large, beaten (1 piece)

Sea salt (1/4 teaspoon)

Vanilla extract (1 teaspoon)

Butter, grass-fed (1/2 cup)

Cinnamon (2 teaspoons)

Maple sugar, granulated (3/4 cup)

Coconut oil, for greasing

Directions:

1. Set the oven at 350 degrees to preheat. Meanwhile, grease a cookie sheet with the coconut oil.
2. In a small bowl, mix the butter and sugar together. Beat in the egg before adding the vanilla, sea salt, cinnamon, and baking powder. Stir in the flour and raisins.
3. Use plastic wrap to cover the mixture. Place in the refrigerator for about two hours to set.
4. Form one-inch rolls out of the chilled cookie mixture. Lay each roll on the cookie sheet and top with a raisin.
5. Place in the oven to bake for about ten minutes. Serve and enjoy.

Chapter 8:
The Best Foods For Thyroid Health

Various hormones are produced by your thyroid. These hormones perform regulatory functions that affect your metabolism, heart rate, body temperature, energy levels, blood pressure, and mood. When the become compromised, resulting in various disorders. Thankfully, there are a number of thyroid-friendly foods you can eat to give your butterfly-shaped gland a boost. You can improve thyroid function when you compliment your medication with balanced nutrition from healthy foods.

1. Beans

Improper thyroid function can make you feel lacking in energy. You can count on beans to provide you the sustained energy you need, especially since they are not expensive and you can incorporate them in many different dishes. Beans are rich sources of complex carbohydrates, proteins, fiber, vitamins, minerals, and antioxidants. Choose from among the different varieties of beans, and use them as starter ingredients for your stews, soups, salads, side dishes, and entrees.

2. Dairy

Studies have identified thyroid disorder associated diseases (including Hashimoto's disease as well as heartburn and other gut issues) as being connected to the lowering of vitamin D levels in the body. For this reason, it is wise to consume vitamin D-rich fortified milk as well as probiotic-rich yogurt to help improve your thyroid function.

3. Fish

Tuna, salmon, trout, sardines, and other fatty fish are rich sources of omega-3 fats, making them a great addition to your dishes. Their omega-3 fat content helps reduce your risk for heart disease, particularly the kind triggered by increased cholesterol levels as a result of poor thyroid function. Omega-3 fatty acids are also known to be effective against inflammation. Moreover, fish contains high amounts of selenium (found in high amounts in your thyroid), another nutrient that helps fight inflammation.

4. Fresh Fruits and Vegetables

Gaining weight is one of the symptoms of poor thyroid function, especially in the early stages. To help you manage your weight, eat fresh fruits and vegetables, which contain low amounts of calories, yet still satiate your appetite. As much as possible, include fruits (such as blueberries and cherries) and vegetables (green peppers and sweet potatoes) in every meal. They contain high levels of heart disease-fighting antioxidants. You may have to steer clear of broccoli, cabbage, and other cruciferous vegetables, however, since they can prevent your thyroid from absorbing iodine (an important nutrient that helps your thyroid to function normally).

5. Nuts

Nuts are handy snack items that do not only taste great and make you feel full; they are also good sources of the mineral selenium, which is another nutrient that helps in proper thyroid function. Add macadamia nuts (a small handful), hazelnuts (a small handful), and Brazil nuts (one to two pieces) to your stir-fry and salad dishes – small amounts go a long way in helping you get your daily recommended amount of nutrients.

6. Seaweed

Seaweed contains high amounts of iodine, which is essential in the proper functioning of your thyroid gland. Include dulse, wakame, nori, and other forms of seaweed in your salads, soups, and sushi to increase your intake of iodine, which is used in producing your thyroid hormones. Further, consuming seaweed allows you to benefit from the vitamins (A, C, E, B, and K), calcium, and fiber it contains. Just make sure to consult your doctor about increasing your intake of iodine, especially if you are already taking iodine supplements – too much can actually make your thyroid problem worse.

7. Whole Grains

One of the common symptoms of poor thyroid function is constipation, which you can remedy with a diet that includes whole grain foods (bread, rice, cereal, and pasta). These food items are all rich in fiber, which helps regulate your bowel movement. It is important to note, however, that fiber can potentially block the absorption of thyroid hormones (synthetic) that you may be taking. You will have to take them a number of hours prior to or following a fiber-rich meal.

Chapter 9:
Vital Nutrients For Thyroid Health

In order for your thyroid gland to be able to function properly, you have to make sure that you are getting the exact vitamins as well as minerals it needs. The way hormones work in the body is unique in each individual, so it would be best to ensure that you consume all of the nutrients that help improve thyroid function, in case you have any deficiencies in those areas.

To help you give your thyroid a boost, make sure to take these highly valuable nutrients:

1. Antioxidants and B Vitamins

You may already know that antioxidants play an important role in fighting off the effects of oxidative stress, namely the aging process as well as a number of degenerative diseases. Together with selenium and iodine, vitamins A (beta-carotene), C, and E aid your thyroid gland in combating oxidative stress, which is associated with hyperthyroidism.

With hyperthyroidism, your thyroid works overtime and ends up using more than the normal amount of oxygen. This results in an increase of by-products that cause damage to your cells. To help prevent the destructive domino effect of oxidative stress, it is recommended that you take antioxidants. Meanwhile, B vitamins (B6, B3, and B2) will help your thyroid produce certain thyroid hormones (namely T4).

2. Copper, Iron, and Zinc

For your thyroid gland to function properly, it also needs these three important trace metals. It requires copper for the production of the Thyroid Stimulating Hormone (TSH) as well as the maintenance of T4 (Thyroxine, the thyroid hormone that regulates your cholesterol levels) production. Furthermore, a number of research studies have indicated that not having enough copper may result in your thyroid disorder being complicated by issues with heart function as well as elevated cholesterol levels.

Iron deficiency can also cause your thyroid to function improperly. In order for thyroid imbalance (due to iodine deficiency) to be corrected, there is also a need to replace iron. Meanwhile, reduced zinc levels can cause your thyroid hormones (namely TSH, T4, and T3 or Triiodothyronine) to decrease in their amounts as well. As shown by research studies, a decrease in thyroid hormone production can result from a zinc deficiency that is due to either an overactive (hyperthyroidism) or underactive (hypothyroidism) thyroid.

3. Iodine

In the case of trace elements involved in thyroid function, iodine is considered to be the most important. Iodine provides the basic components that your thyroid needs to manufacture the hormones that support your bodily tissues, the most important of which are T4 and T3. Eating foods that are rich in iodine can help improve your iodine levels to thyroid-friendly amounts.

4. Selenium

In a number of ways, your thyroid cannot do without selenium. During times of stress, the element, which acts through the enzymes it is contained in, gives protection to your thyroid gland through detoxification, attacking oxidative, chemical, and even social stressors. Together with certain proteins, selenium also aids in regulating the production of hormones, specifically in the conversion of T4 into T3 (more accessible form).

Both these selenium-containing enzymes and selenium-based proteins support regular metabolism as well as maintenance of thyroid hormone levels in the blood and tissues and organs (brain, kidney, and liver). Moreover, selenium also controls as well as replenishes your body's iodine levels.

Chapter 10:
How Thyroid Disorders Are Diagnosed

The Mimic: Hyperthyroidism

Higher than normal levels of thyroid hormones can lead to the disorder called hyperthyroidism, which can closely resemble other health disorders. This is what makes hyperthyroidism hard to diagnose, especially with the wide variety of symptoms and signs it causes.

Signs and symptoms: These include fatigue and muscle weakness; increased appetite; sudden weight loss; trouble sleeping; changes in bowel movement frequency; irritability, anxiety, and nervousness; menstrual pattern changes; increased heat sensitivity; sweating; hair becoming brittle and fine; thinning of the skin; fine trembling of the fingers and hands (tremor); rapid heartbeat, irregular heartbeat, or heart palpitations; and enlargement of the thyroid gland.

Diagnosis: In the diagnosis of thyroid disorders, specifically hyperthyroidism, measurement of the TSH (Thyroid Stimulating Hormone) is considered the most useful blood test. A low TSH count means that the thyroid hormones found in the blood are higher than normal, indicating that you have hyperthyroidism. Keep in mind that these tests are old, and are not 100% accurate all of the time. Multiple tests may be necessary to get a firm diagnosis.

The Silent Worker: Hypothyroidism

Having too little of thyroid hormones, on the other hand, characterizes the thyroid disorder referred to as hypothyroidism. It is actually considered a common problem, and what makes hypothyroidism difficult to diagnose as well is that it can go unnoticed for many years before you recognize that you have it.

Signs and symptoms: Signs and symptoms of hypothyroidism include unexplained weight gain; weakness, aches, stiffness, and tenderness of the muscles; increased cold sensitivity; heavier or irregular menstruation; constipation; higher blood cholesterol levels; swelling, stiffness, or pain in the joints; fatigue; slower heart rate; memory impairment; hoarseness; thinning of the hair; dry skin; puffiness of the face; and depression.

Diagnosis: As in the case of hypothyroidism, blood tests are also relied upon in diagnosing hypothyroidism. They include measuring your TSH (Thyroid Stimulating Hormone) levels as well as Thyroxine (T4) levels. You have a thyroid gland that is underactive if your blood tests show low T4 levels and high TSH levels (your pituitary gland makes more TSH than usual in its attempt to encourage your thyroid gland to make more thyroid hormones). Keep in mind that once again, these tests are old, and are not 100% accurate all of the time. Multiple tests may be necessary to get a firm diagnosis.

Other Diagnostic Tests

T4 Blood Test: High levels of T4 in the blood may be an indicator of an overactive thyroid (hyperthyroidism), whereas low levels of T4 could indicate that you have hypothyroidism.

T3 Blood Test: As in the case of the diagnostic test based on your T4 levels, a high T3 level could be an indicator of hyperthyroidism while a lower T3 count could mean that you have hypothyroidism.

Nuclear Thyroid Scan: This nuclear scanning of your thyroid gland involves swallowing radioactive iodine in small amounts, or getting your bloodstream injected with 99m-technetium (a material that is similar to iodine). Your thyroid is then subjected to imaging studies in order to reveal where the radioactivity is localized. If there is an increased uptake of iodine or technetium, then hyperthyroidism is diagnosed. Hypothyroidism is indicated, on the other hand, if there is decreased iodine or technetium uptake.

Chapter 11:
Medical Treatments For Thyroid Disorders

A number of medical treatments are used by mainstream medicine to manage thyroid disorders. It is important that you consult your doctor about any side effects that are caused by your prescribed medication, and make sure that you follow proper dosing and schedule.

Medical Treatments for Hyperthyroidism

1. Beta-blockers

To manage hyperthyroidism, beta-blockers prevent your body from responding to the thyroid disorder, resulting in the reduction of a fast heart rate as well as agitation, nervousness, and tremor. Prescribed in tablet form or as intravenous preparation, beta-blocker tablets are ideal for cases with mild to moderate symptoms. On the other hand, IV preparation is more appropriate for those with more severe symptoms, such as a thyrotoxic crisis. It is important to note, as their name implies, beta-blockers simply block your body's response to hyperthyroidism.

2. Iodide

Administered in the form of strong iodine or Lugol's solution, the iodide medication effectively prevents the thyroid hormone produced by your overactive thyroid from being released. An anti-thyroid drug is used as a partner of iodide, since the latter can cause a higher production of thyroid hormones, which only makes your hyperthyroidism worse. Feelings of nausea as well as having a metallic taste in your mouth are the common side effects of the iodide medical treatment.

3. Methimazole

Excluding pregnant women who are in their first trimester, most people with hyperthyroidism prefer the anti-thyroid drug methimazole. It works by blocking the production of thyroid hormones.

4. Propylthiouracil

Propylthiouracil is another anti-thyroid drug that works by inhibiting the synthesis of thyroid hormones. You may feel its therapeutic effects several months into your medical treatment, although this is considered faster compared to methimazole. You may take propylthiouracil even if you are pregnant (but only in the first trimester stage), and if you are found to be intolerant to thimazole medications. You may experience an itchy rash (a mild side effect that is common) when taking propylthiouracil, or you might have a high fever due to a reduction of white blood cells (serious side effect that is rare), in which you should your doctor right away.

5. Radioactive Iodine Therapy

Requiring the expertise of either a specialist in nuclear medicine or an endocrinologist, this therapy involves swallowing radioactive iodine (different from that used in diagnostic tests) to treat hyperthyroidism. Radioactive iodine therapy causes your thyroid gland to become smaller after getting it scarred several months into the treatment.

Medical Treatments for Hypothyroidism

1. L-thyroxine

The different forms of L-thyroxine (synthetic T4), such as Levoxyl, Unithroid, Synthroid, Levothroid, and Tirsosint, are considered the mainstays of hypothyroidism therapy that involves replacement of thyroid hormones. L-thyroxine works by being converted by your bodily tissues into the active, more accessible L-triiodothyronine (synthetic T3). Having an outstanding safety record, it rarely triggers side effects.

2. Triiodothyronine

Lasting less time in your bloodstream than L-thyroxine does, triiodothronine is hardly used on its own in thyroid hormone replacement therapy. It may treat hypothyroidism symptoms when used with L-thyroxine, especially when the latter works poorly when used alone. Elderly people and heart disease patients are discouraged from taking triiodothyronine medications due to their ability to cause too much of a rapid increase of triiodothyronine levels.

3. Thyroid extract

The thyroid extract is actually a pig's thyroid gland in dry, powdered form. Because there is no hormone purification involved, resulting in inconsistent amounts of T3 and T4, thyroid extracts are not recommended in replacement therapy of thyroid hormones.

Chapter 12:
How The Thyroid Works & Affects The Whole Body

The Workings of Your Thyroid

Inconspicuous. Your thyroid gland lies inside your neck, right on top of the Adam's apple, in the shape of a butterfly. But what is more interesting to know is the fact that this unassuming gland can have such a dramatic impact on how your body carries out its duties.

Instrument of Mayhem. Thyroid hormones are produced by your thyroid gland, and they take care of several functions that include regulating your heartbeat, metabolism, and temperature. When the levels of these hormones are not stabilized, however, that is when your body gets negatively affected in a number of ways. Things go haywire when the thyroid becomes overactive or underactive. Too little thyroid hormones get produced when your thyroid works sluggishly. On the other hand, if it works overtime, then it manufactures too much thyroid hormones.

Cause of Chaos. Experts are still divided with regards to the root of it all, but they have pinpointed nutritional deficiencies, genetics, stress, autoimmune attacks, environmental toxins, and even pregnancy as possible causes of a thyroid gone wild. What makes the thyroid gland have such a big impact on your body is the fact that its hormones reaches so many parts in your body.

How Your Body Is Affected by Your Thyroid

Here are the ways in which your thyroid affects your entire body when it is not functioning properly:

1. Flutters and jitters.

A thyroid disorder can cause you to feel all fluttery because of the heart palpitations. You either feel as though your heart itself is skipping by one or two beats, or it is beating too fast or too hard, and these feelings are felt in the chest area or in the pulse points of your neck or throat. These fluttery feelings may be due to the excess thyroid hormones in your system that result in hyperthyroidism.

Feeling all anxious and jittery is another sign of hyperthyroidism. The increase in thyroid hormone levels can cause your body to go into an all-systems-go mode, which makes it difficult for you to feel relaxed.

2. Feeling down and out.

Feeling sad or depressed is a sign of hypothyroidism, which is a disorder that results when too little hormones are produced by your thyroid. When this gland goes into underactive mode, the serotonin level in your brain is affected, causing your mood to dip.

Hypothyroidism can also cause you to feel tired and lacking in energy. Your muscles are not able to receive the go signal from your cells and bloodstream, since there are not enough thyroid hormones traveling through them. You might then feel too tired to get up in the morning, even if you have had proper sleep the night before.

3. Altered appetite, weight, and bowels.

One of the signs of hyperthyroidism is an increase in your appetite, causing you to always feel hungry. This has a surprising positive spin, though; even if you constantly eat, you will not gain weight due to the "hyper" end of this disorder of the thyroid gland. Meanwhile, hypothyroidism can wreak havoc on the way you smell and taste food, which results in weight gain.

Constipation is another symptom of hypothyroidism. Because of the disruption caused by the decreased amount of thyroid hormones produced, your digestive processes can experience a slowdown. On the other hand, over activity of the thyroid gland (hyperthyroidism) can cause you to have diarrhea or experience an increase in the number of your bowel movements.

4. Unexpected bodily changes.

Having the chills is one of the bodily changes associated with an underactive thyroid. Hypothyroidism can cause your cells to burn less energy, resulting in a slowdown of your system. Less body heat is released when less energy is burned, causing you to feel cold. Hyperthyroidism, on the other hand, makes the cells in your body that produce energy go into overdrive. This is the reason individuals suffering from an overactive thyroid sweat too much or feel too warm.

Dry, itchy skin is another common symptom associated with an underactive thyroid. Because too little of the thyroid hormones are produced, your metabolism slows down and decreases your ability to perspire. This leads to your skin lacking the proper amount of moisture it needs, causing it to turn flaky and dry. For the same reason, your nails may develop rides and get brittle.

When you have an underactive thyroid, you may also experience having brittle and dry hair that falls out and easily breaks. Reduction in your thyroid hormone levels can hinder the complete cycle of your hair growth. A large number of follicles go into resting mode and as a result, results in the loss of your hair strands – not just on your head, but sometimes also throughout your entire body. On the other hand, hyperthyroidism can cause your hair to thin out in numbers.

You might find yourself working out too hard or stubbing your toe, and then feel pain afterwards. In the case of hypothyroidism, however, you may feel some sudden tingling, a mysterious numbing sensation, or an actual painful feeling in your hands, arms, feet, and legs. In the long run, the decrease in thyroid hormone levels causes your nerves to get damaged. This prompts your brain as well as spinal cord to send signals all over your body, resulting in your unexpected twinges and tingles.

5. Skyrocketing blood pressure and cholesterol levels.

An increase in blood pressure levels can be another symptom of a thyroid problem, both hypothyroidism and hyperthyroidism. If your thyroid problem has to do with an underactive thyroid, you have an increased risk for hypertension.

Hypothyroidism can also cause you to have higher levels of bad cholesterol, even with the help of medication, exercise, and diet. This can lead to enlargement of the heart, heart failure, and other heart problems.

6. Sleeplessness and fuzzy feelings.

If you find yourself wanting to sleep as much as you can, then it could be due to your thyroid gland being sluggish. This leads to the slowing down of the different functions performed by your body, causing the latter to think that sleeping in the daytime is a great thing to do.

If, on the other hand, you are having difficulty in going to sleep, then it could be attributed to an overactive thyroid. This condition causes you to experience anxiety and an increased pulse rate, resulting in you having a hard time sleeping, or easily waking up during the night. Getting deprived of enough sleep plus having a thyroid problem (hypothyroidism or hyperthyroidism) can also cause you to become forgetful and feel fuzzy.

Conclusion

Thank you again for downloading this book!

I hope this book was able to help you learn more about thyroid disorders!

The next step is to put this information to use, and begin improving your thyroid disorder with a change in diet!

Finally, if you enjoyed this book, please take the time to share your thoughts and post a review on Amazon. It'd be greatly appreciated!

Thank you and good luck!